Mindfulness

IS YOUR

SUPERPOWER

Mindfulness IS YOUR SUPER POWER

A Book About Finding Focus and Cultivating Calm

WRITTEN BY
Lauren Stockly,
LCSW, RPT-S, ECMHS, PPSC

ILLUSTRATED BY
Zach Grzeszkowiak

ROCKRIDGE
PRESS

For general information on our other products and services or to obtain technical support, please contact our Customer Care Department within the United States at (866) 744-2665, or outside the United States at (510) 253-0500.

Rockridge Press publishes its books in a variety of electronic and print formats. Some content that appears in print may not be available in electronic books, and vice versa.

Series Designer: Angie Chu
Interior and Cover Designer: Lisa Schreiber
Art Producer: Sara Feinstein
Editor: Sasha Henriques
Production Editor: Dylan Julian
Production Manager: Martin Worthington

Paperback ISBN: 978-1-63878-399-2
eBook ISBN: 978-1-63878-557-6
R0
Printed in China

Ming and Mateo aren't just regular kids—they are best friends with a superpower! Their superpower is called mindfulness. It helps them understand feelings they have inside and better connect to people around them. It also helps them stay calm.

Did you know *you* have a mindfulness superpower, too?

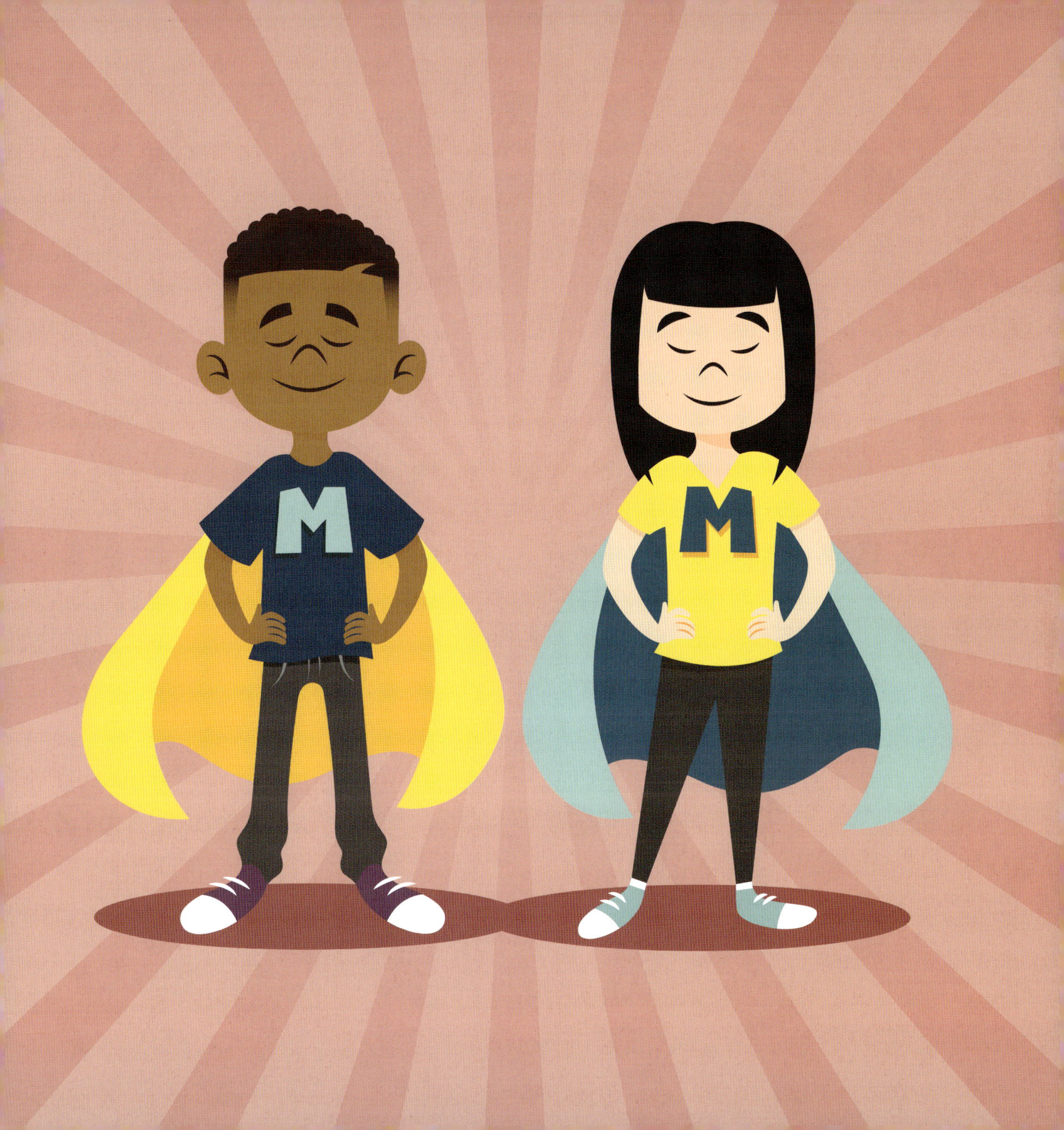
M
M

Sometimes our brains are like messy rooms, with thoughts everywhere. Mindfulness keeps your brain organized so you can learn, play, and feel your best. Activating your power is as easy as focusing on the moment you are in and noticing each of your senses: sight, sound, touch, smell, and taste. Once you are focused on the *here* and *now*, you are being mindful.

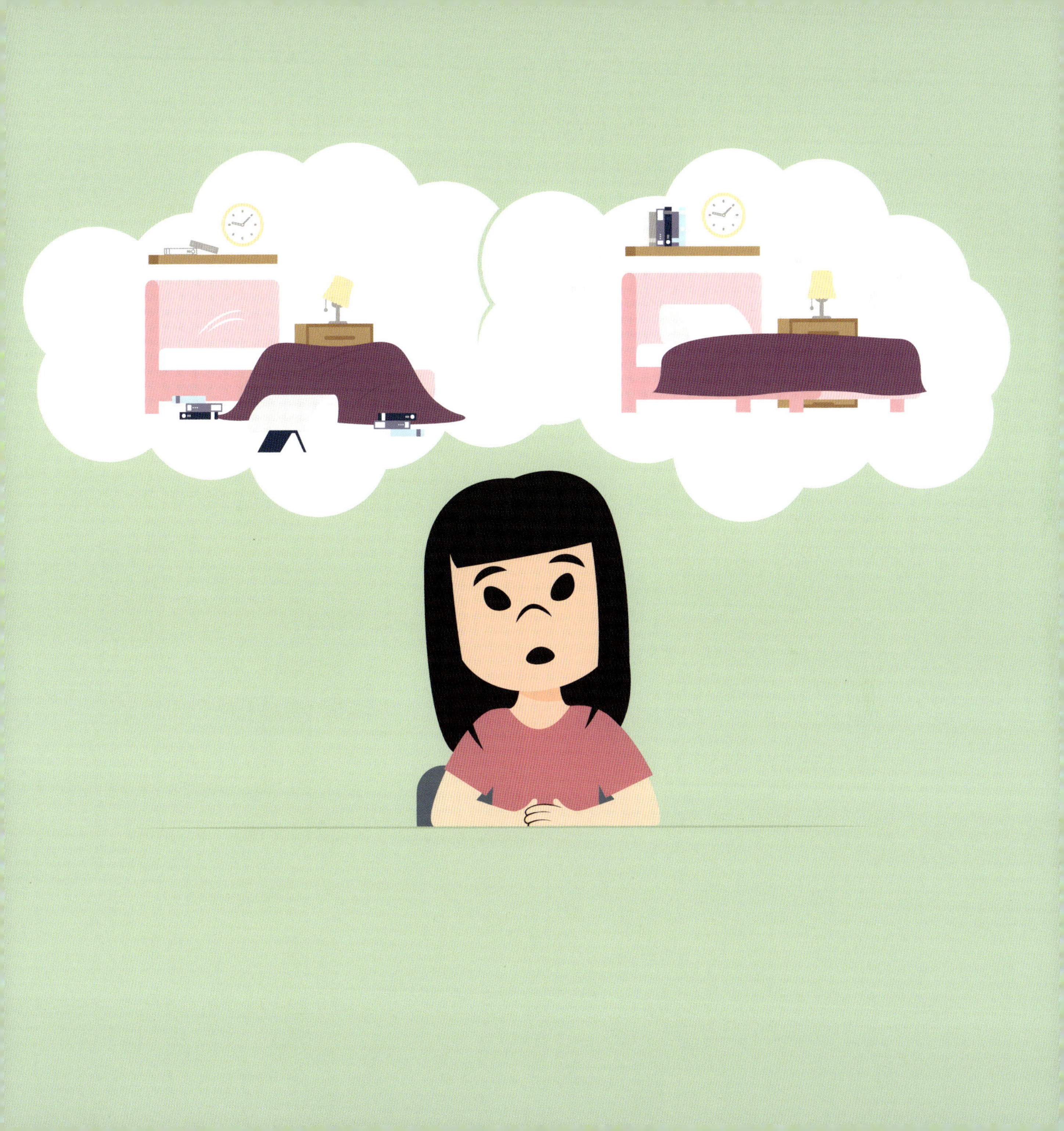

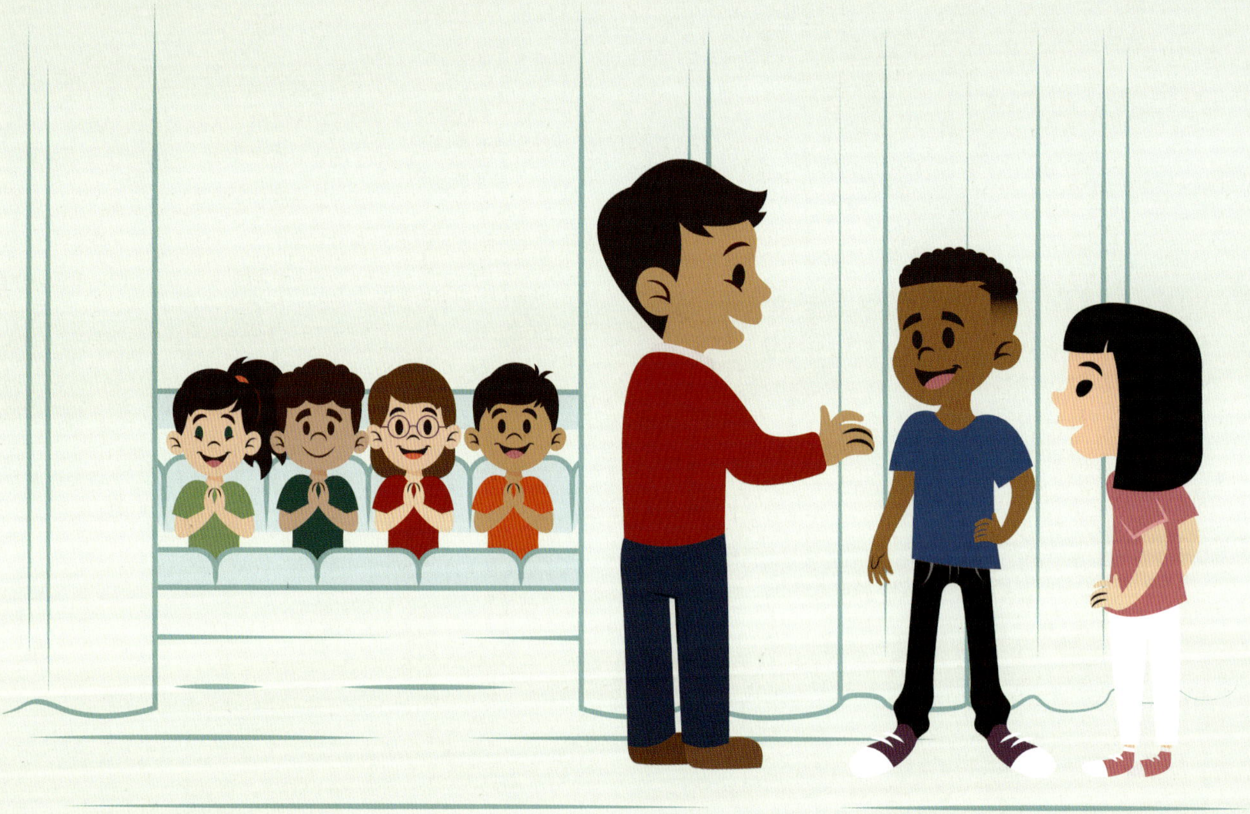

There are many ways to use the amazing power of mindfulness. When Mateo gets nervous in front of a crowd, mindfulness helps him calm down. Listening to the voice of the director keeps him focused.

Why might Mateo have been feeling nervous?

How can paying attention to what is happening in the moment help Mateo feel calm?

On a walk with Ming, Ming's aunt paid attention to the sunlight shining through the trees and the sounds of their footsteps. She told Ming that even when her mind starts to wander, her senses can bring her back and let her focus on where she is.

Which senses did Ming's aunt focus on during their walk?

Look around you now. What are three tiny details you notice?

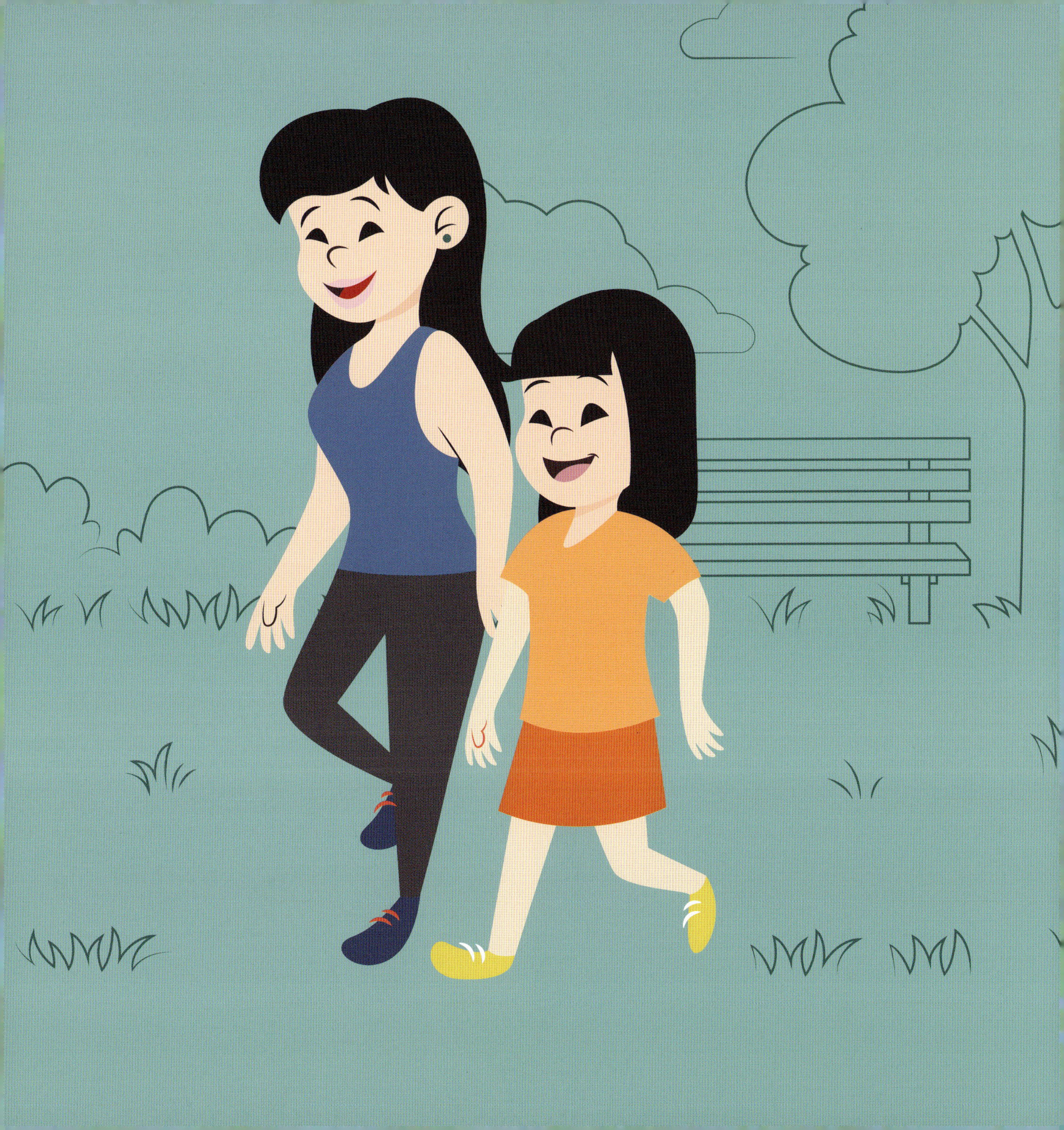

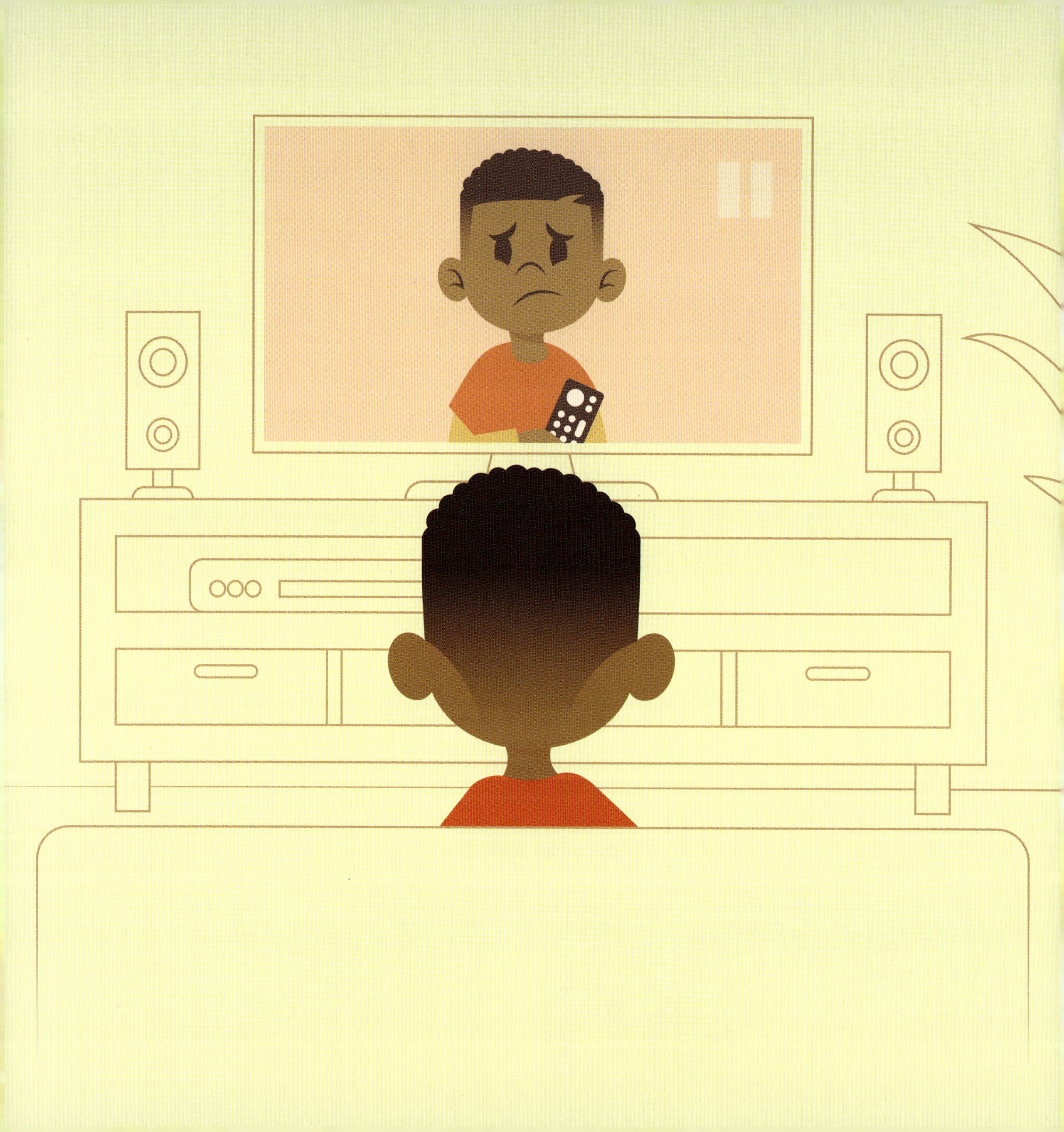

Some feelings are hard or uncomfortable. Mindfulness is like a special "pause" button that gives us time to visit our overwhelming feelings. It's important to make time to care for all our feelings.

Do you think "pressing pause" can help you see your feelings differently?

Can you think of a time when you needed a pause?

You won't always agree with everyone. Some things won't be how you imagined them to be. Mindfulness helps you feel okay when things don't go your way.

Ming and Mateo will show us how they use mindfulness every day.

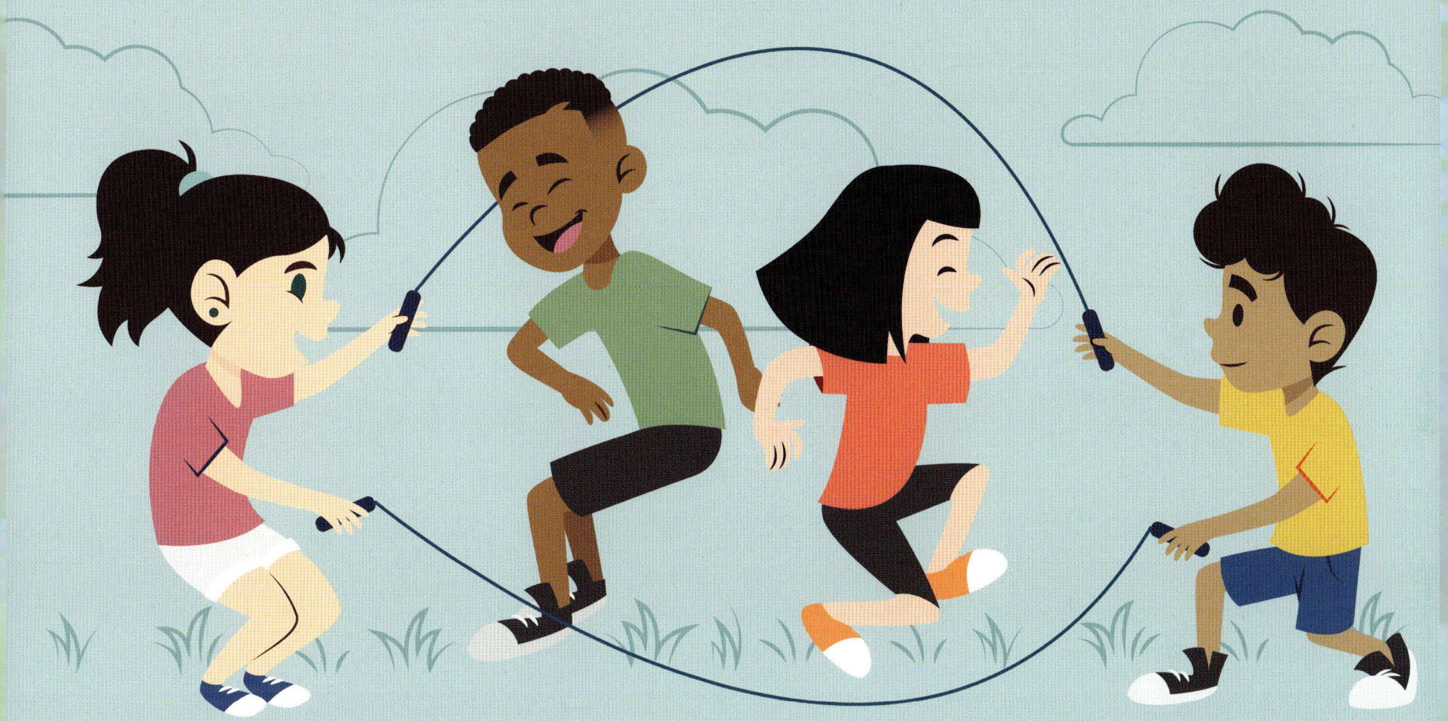

What do you enjoy that someone important to you doesn't enjoy?

What is something new you were glad you tried?

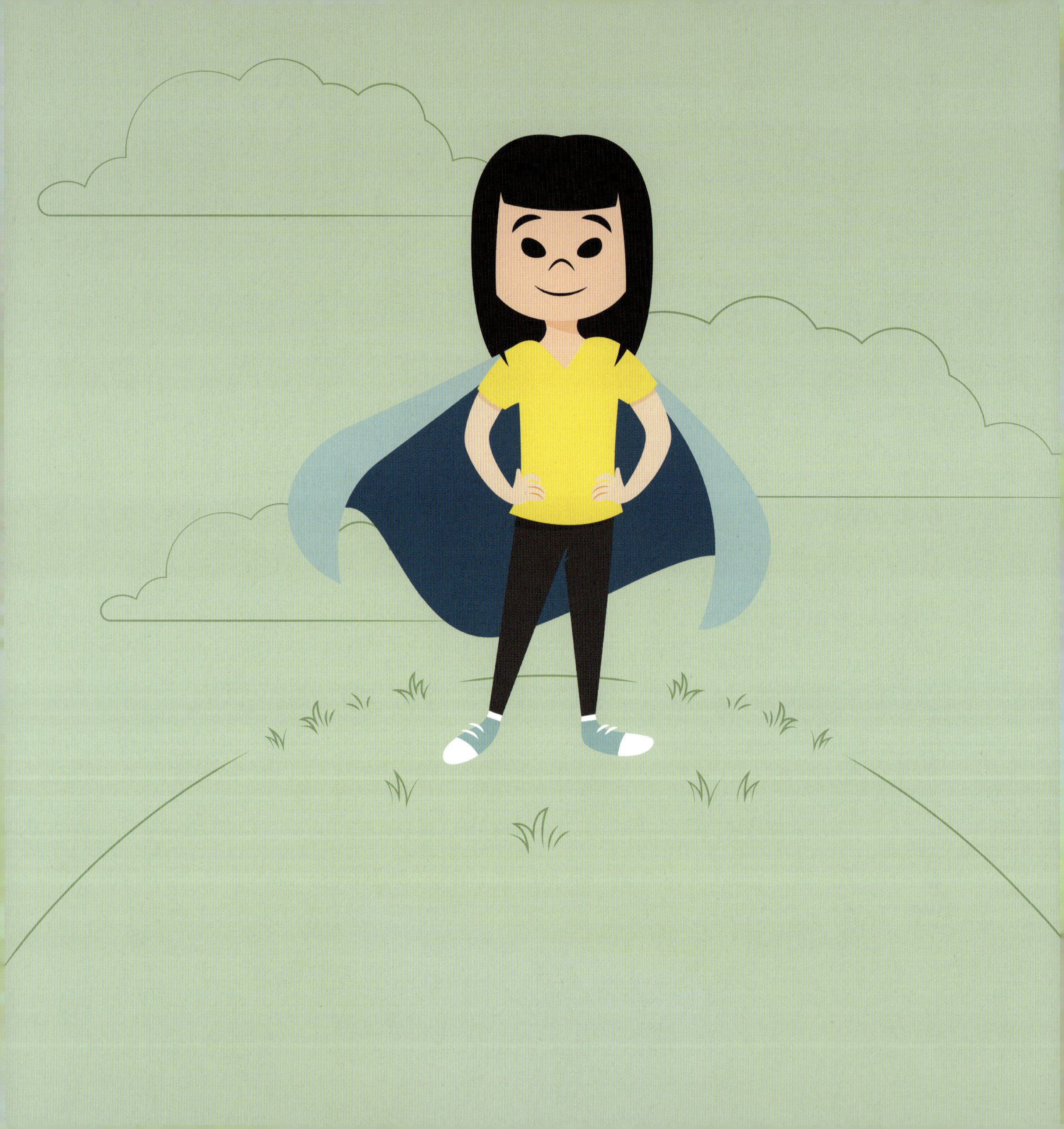

Ming was worried about meeting her teacher. Then she remembered her superhero pose! She stood tall and proud, with her head held high, and focused on the feeling of her feet planted firmly on the floor. Ming took a deep breath. She felt strong and prepared.

Why do you think Ming's superhero pose helped her feel confident?

Do you notice a connection between your body and your feelings?

Mateo wanted to play kickball, but his friend Emmanuel didn't. Instead of losing his temper, Mateo took a mindful moment for himself. When he closed his eyes, he found an angry feeling in his chest. But he could also feel a cool breeze and hear a bird chirping. Focusing on his senses helped Mateo feel calmer. He remembered lots of other fun games he and Emmanuel could play instead.

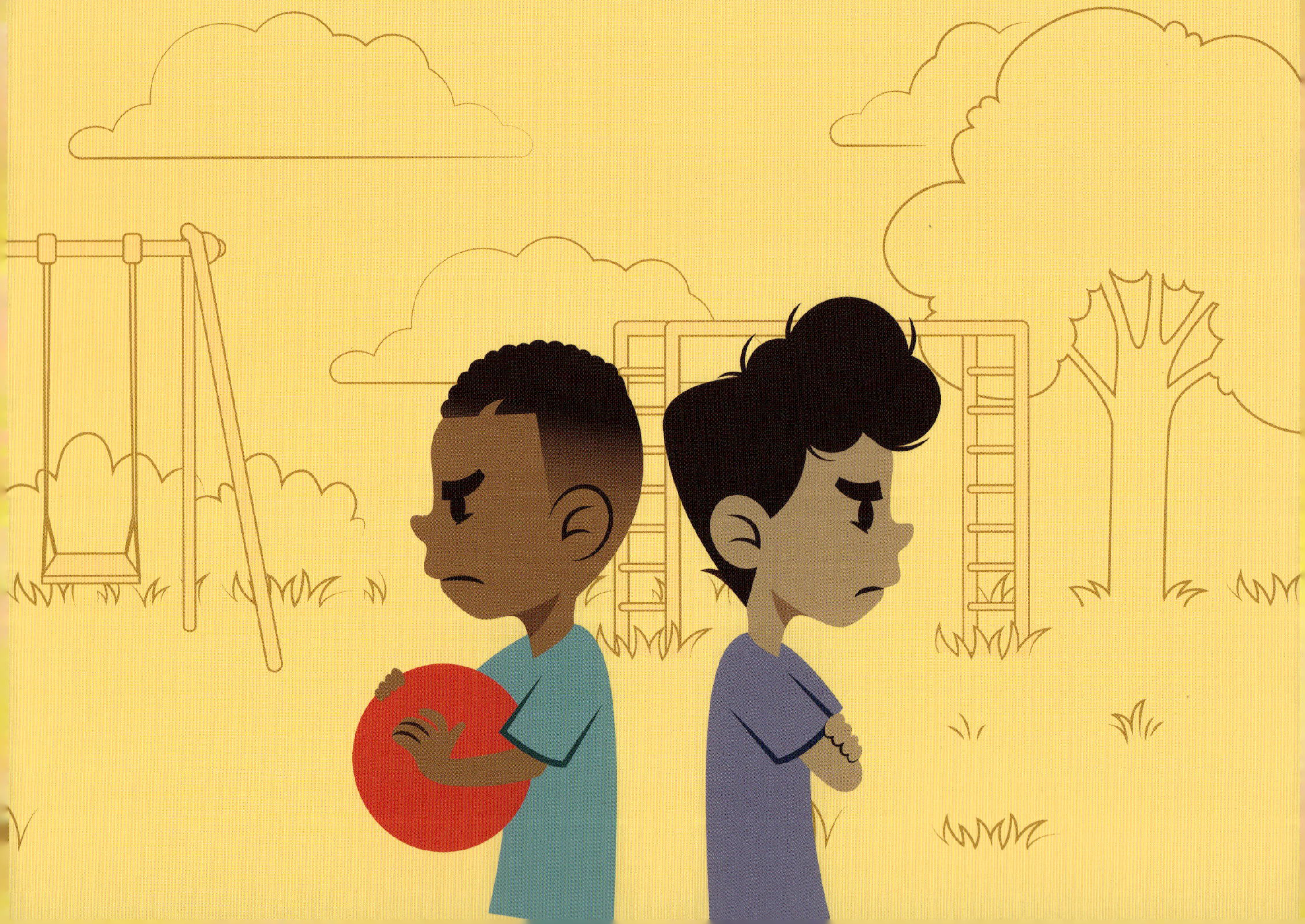

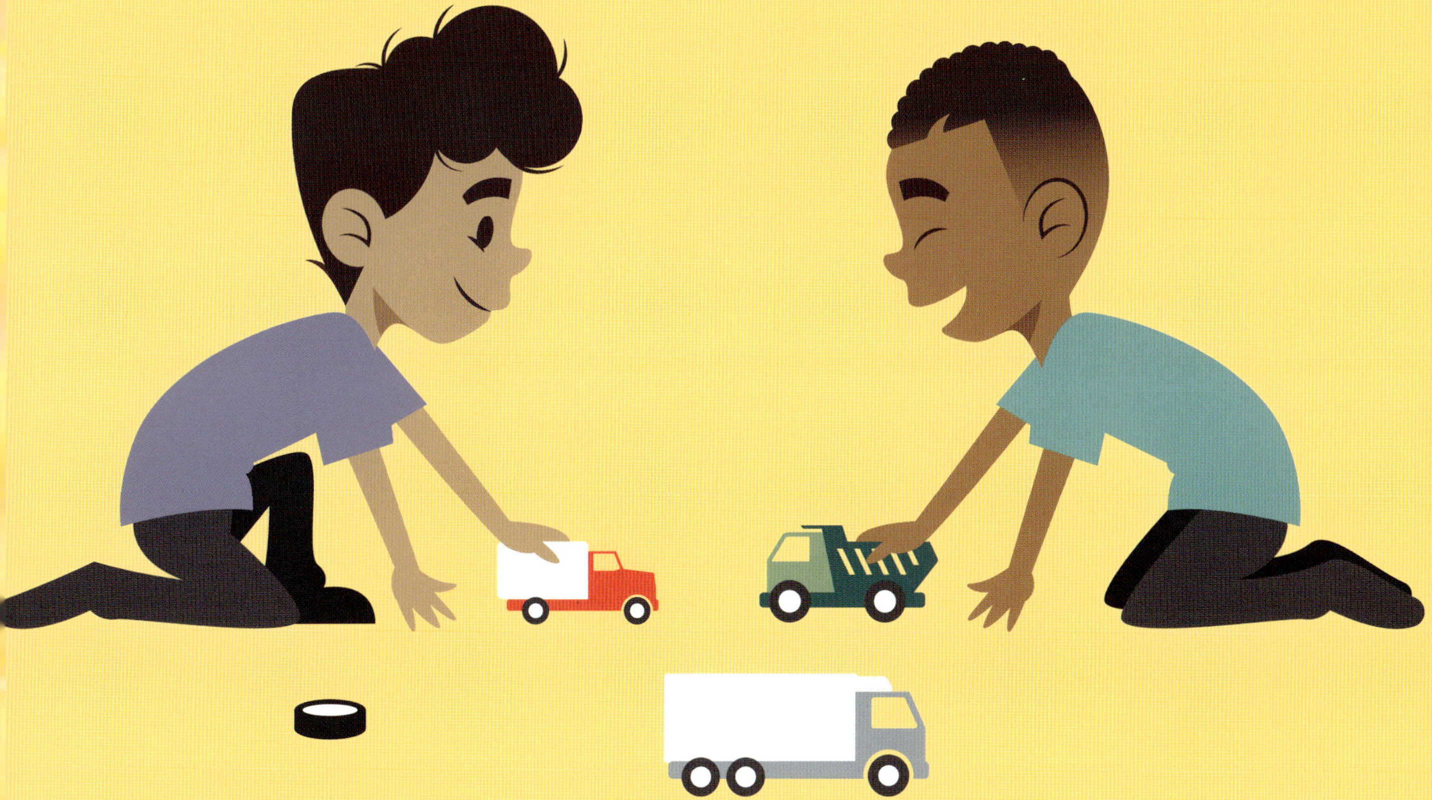

How did Mateo know he needed a mindful moment?

Where do you feel anger in your body?

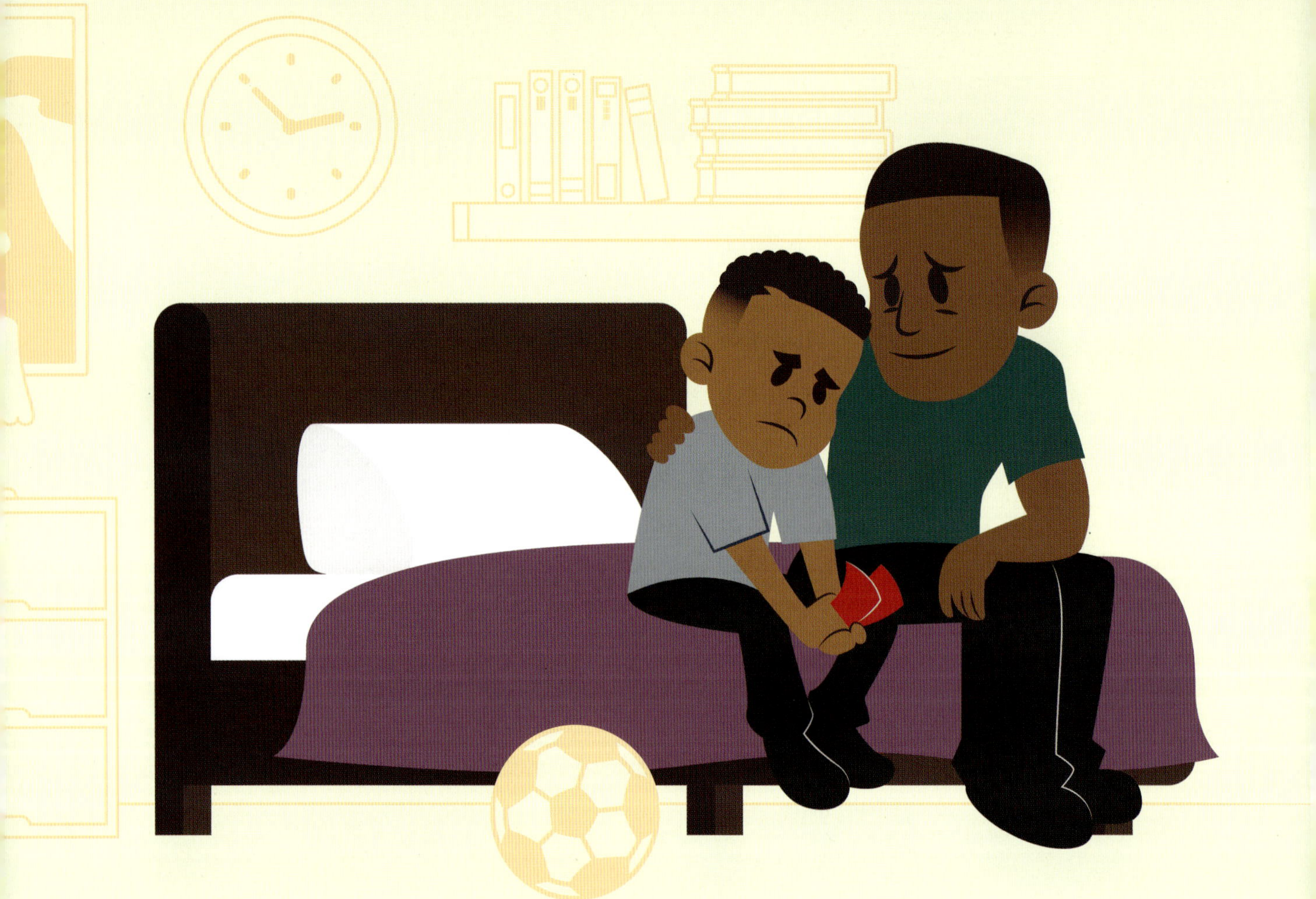

Mateo got upset when the big concert was canceled. He thought pushing his feelings away would make things better, but he only felt worse. He decided to face his feelings with mindfulness and let them in. They were so strong he started to cry. But soon he noticed the disappointment moving along and leaving space for other feelings.

How did mindfulness help Mateo handle his feelings of sadness?

Think about the last time you cried. Did you feel different when you were finished?

Ming taught Grace and Guillermo a great way to be mindful. “Close your eyes. Imagine somewhere safe and calm,” Ming told them. As Grace and Guillermo pictured peaceful places, they felt more and more relaxed.

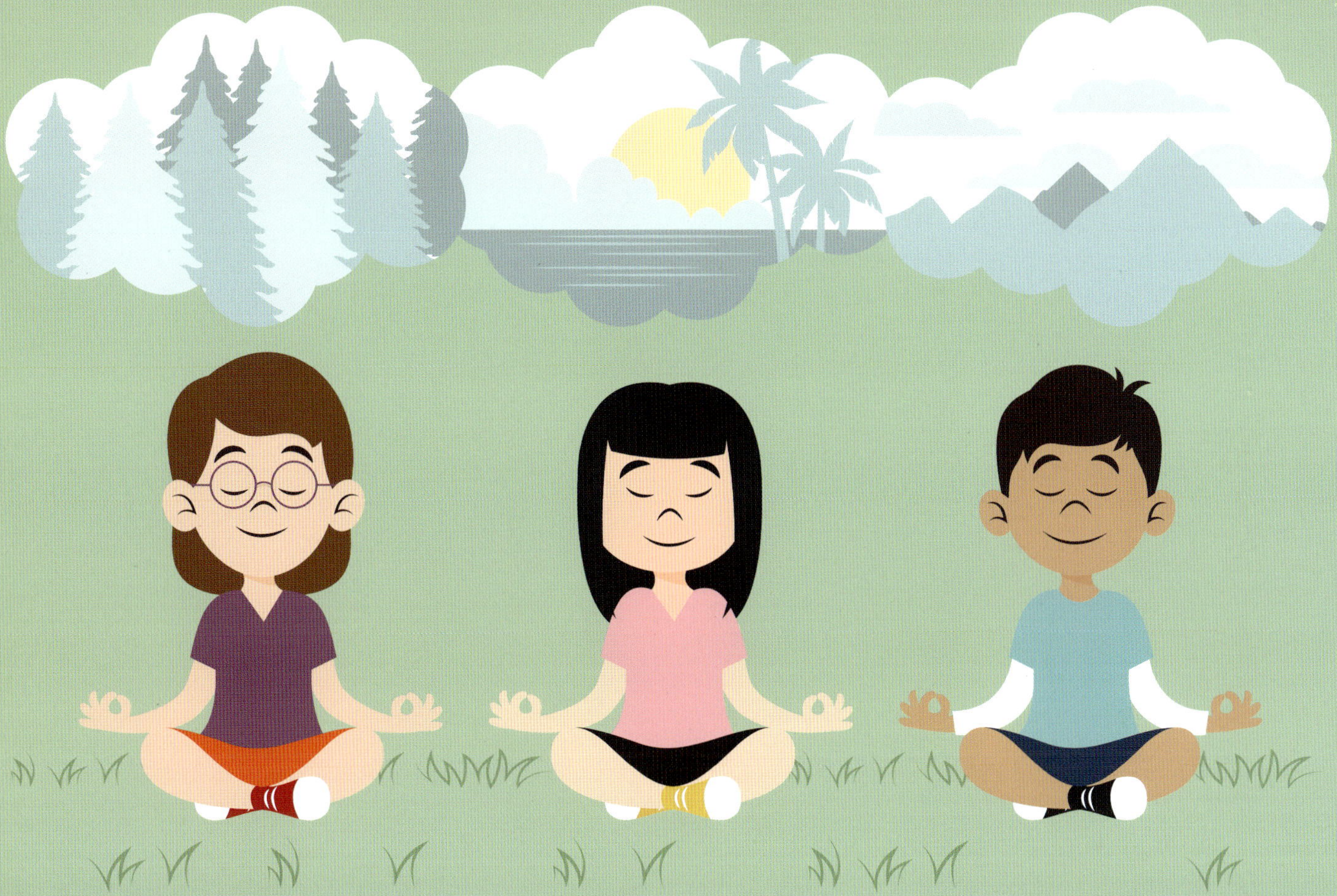

How was Ming able to share her superpower?

Imagine your peaceful place. How does it look, sound, smell, and feel?

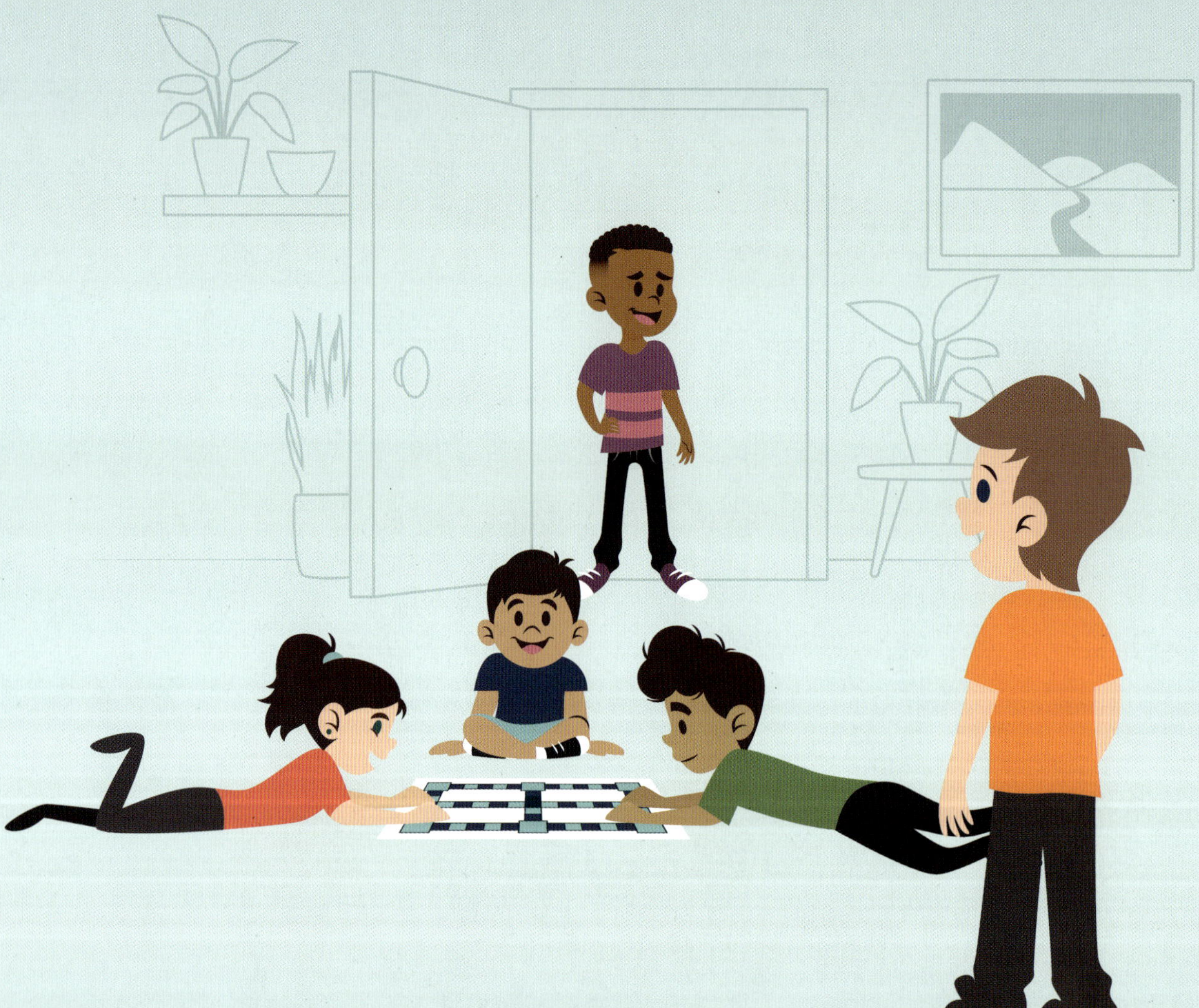

Mateo didn't know why he was nervous, so he used mindfulness to find out. While he focused on the fluttering in his stomach, a thought popped up: "What if no one likes my new shirt?" Mateo knew what the feeling was about. He reminded himself that it didn't matter what anyone else thought. He loved his shirt, and he looked awesome in it!

How did spending time with his anxious feeling help Mateo?

Why is it important to know what is causing our feelings?

Mateo saw that Guillermo was frustrated with math homework. Mateo said to him, "Maybe you can use mindfulness to investigate your feelings like a detective."

Guillermo tried to be curious about his frustration. He noticed that when he didn't know the answers to a math problem, he didn't feel smart. When Guillermo remembered that not knowing all the answers is part of learning, he felt more patient.

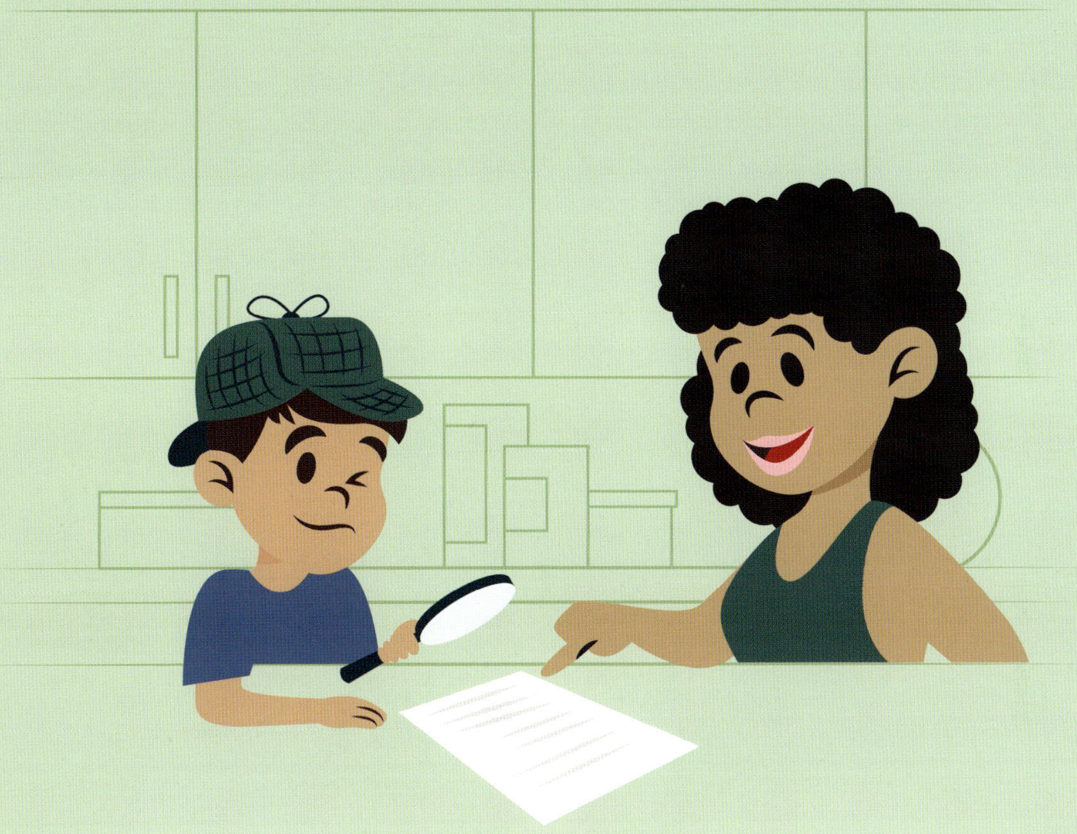

How did learning more about his feeling of frustration help Guillermo?

How could you treat a feeling with curiosity?

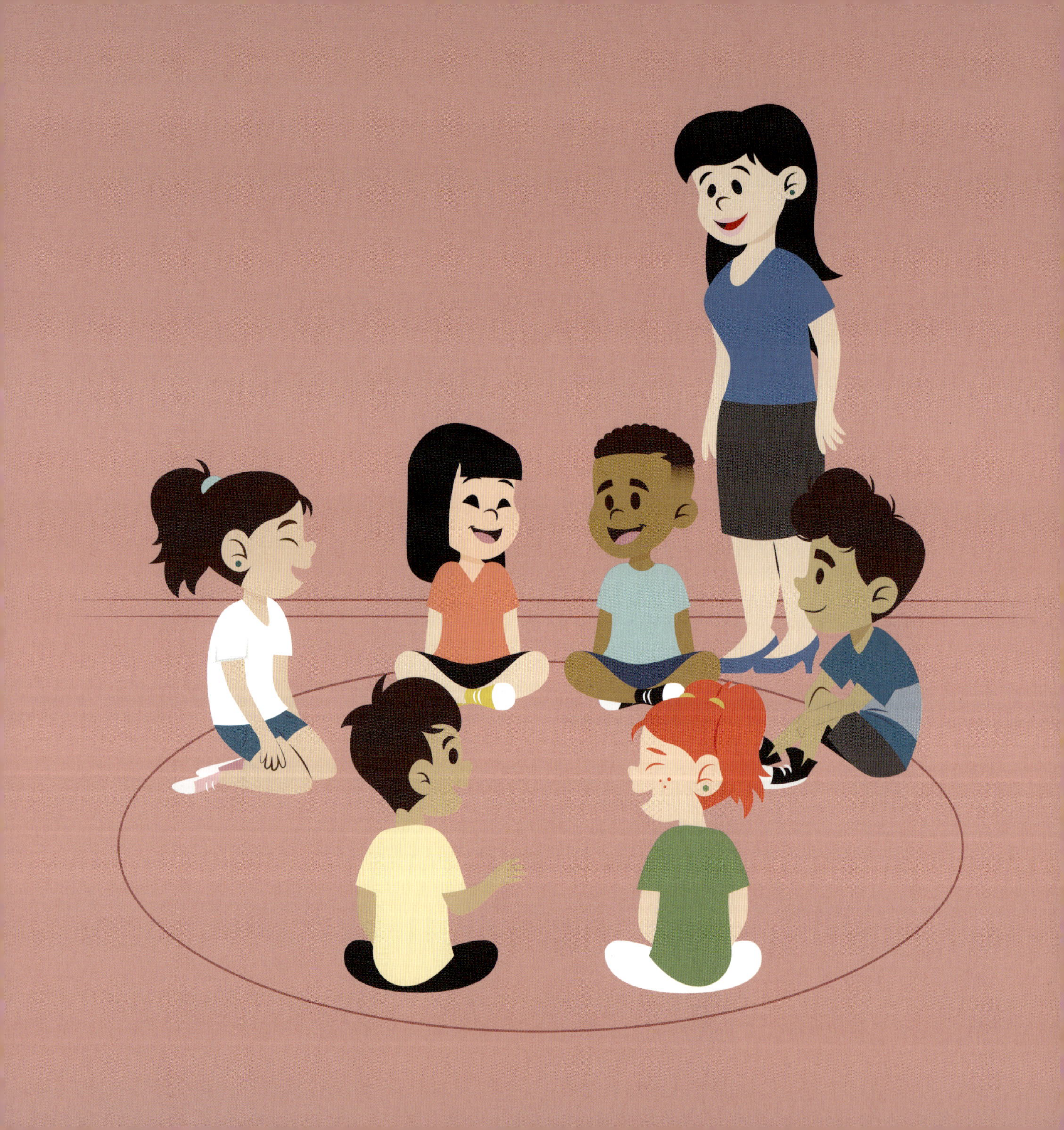

Ming got to lead her classmates in a gratitude circle. As they went around, each person shared something they were grateful for and how it made them feel. Taking time to practice being thankful reminds us of all the things in our lives that make us happy.

How did Ming help her friends remember all the things that make them happy?

What are some ways you can practice being thankful?

Ming's chest ached with sadness when her grandma couldn't come to her birthday party. She knew she couldn't simply stop her feelings, but with mindfulness she could try to accept them. She realized she felt so strongly because she loved her grandma so much. Even uncomfortable feelings deserve to be treated with kindness.

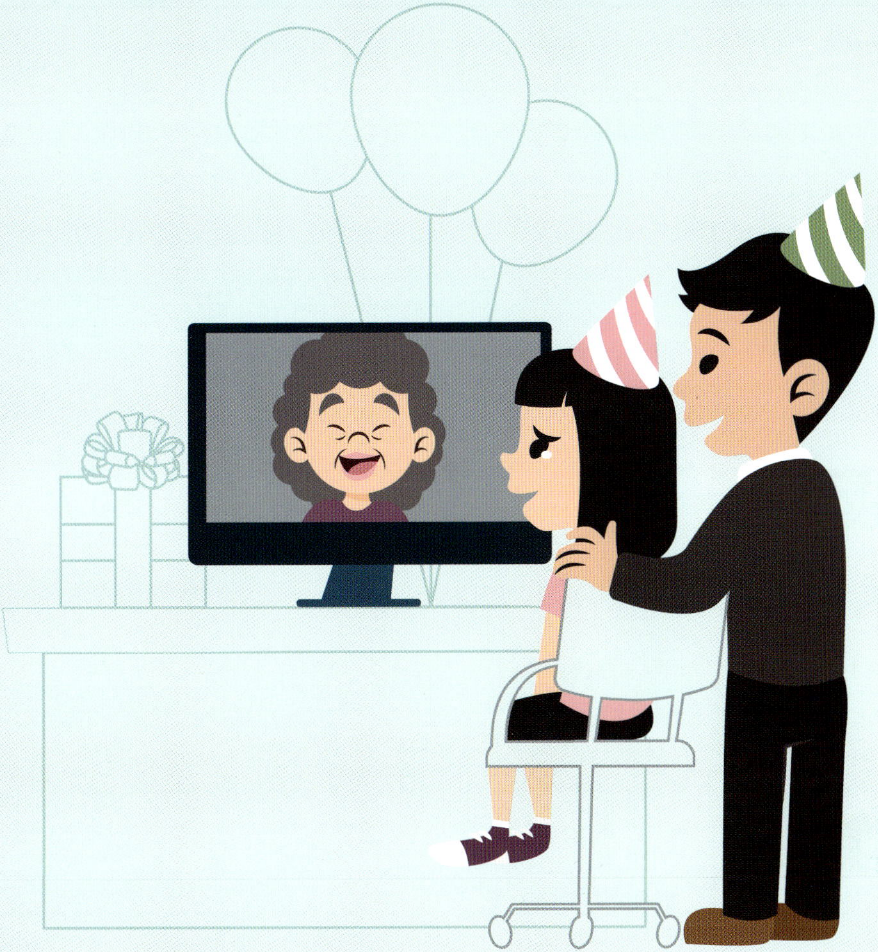

How did Ming use her superpower to figure out where her sadness came from?

The next time you feel sad or angry, how can you treat those feelings with kindness?

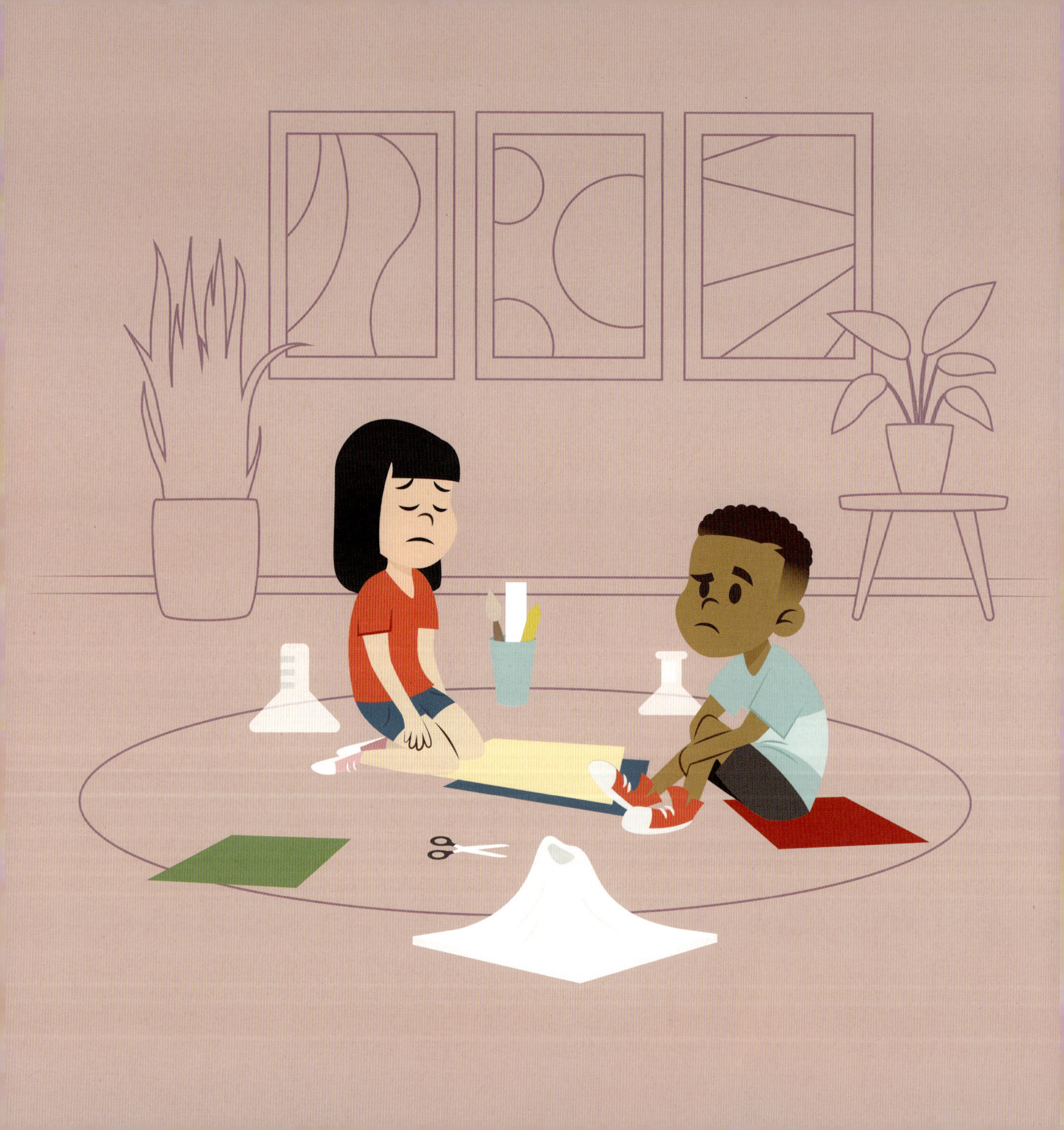

Ming was worried about the science fair, so she greeted the worry to find out why it was there. As she sat with her feelings, she realized they were just reminding her to do her best. Focusing on the moment helped her settle her mind so she could finish her project.

What might have happened to the anxiety if Ming ignored it?

How can you visit with an uncomfortable feeling?

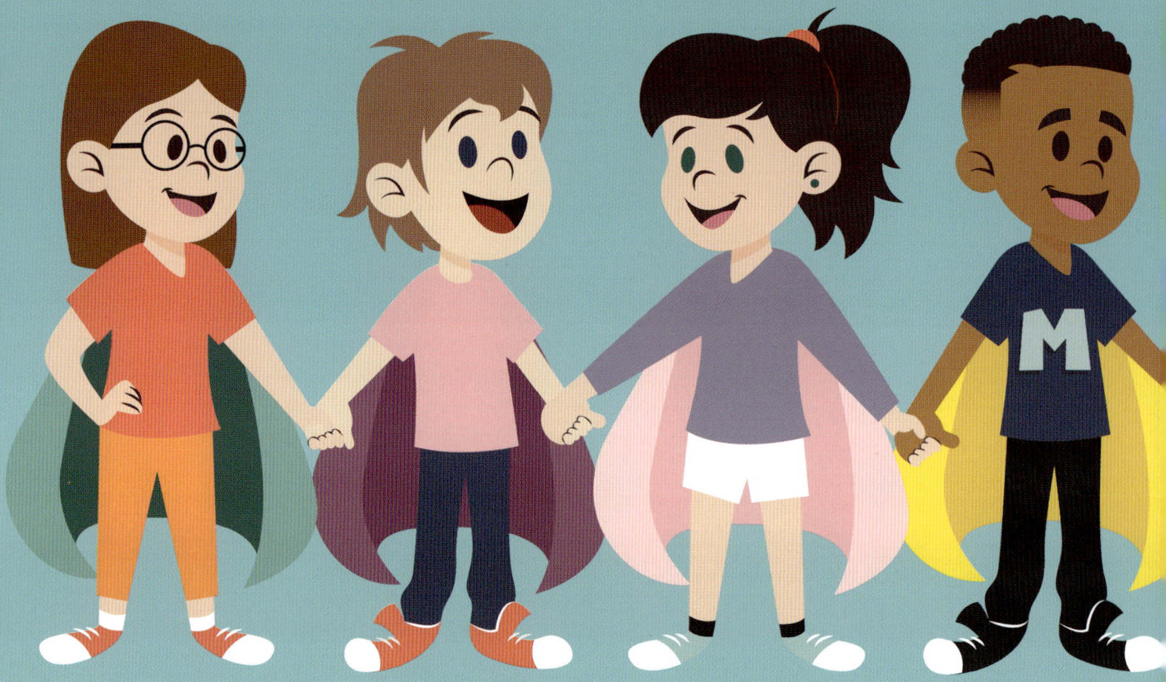

Ming and Mateo use mindfulness to do all sorts of incredible things, like focus better in school, be kinder to others, and stay healthy inside and out. Because they practice their superpower daily, it continues to get stronger.

You now know all about mindfulness, too!
How will *you* use your superpower?

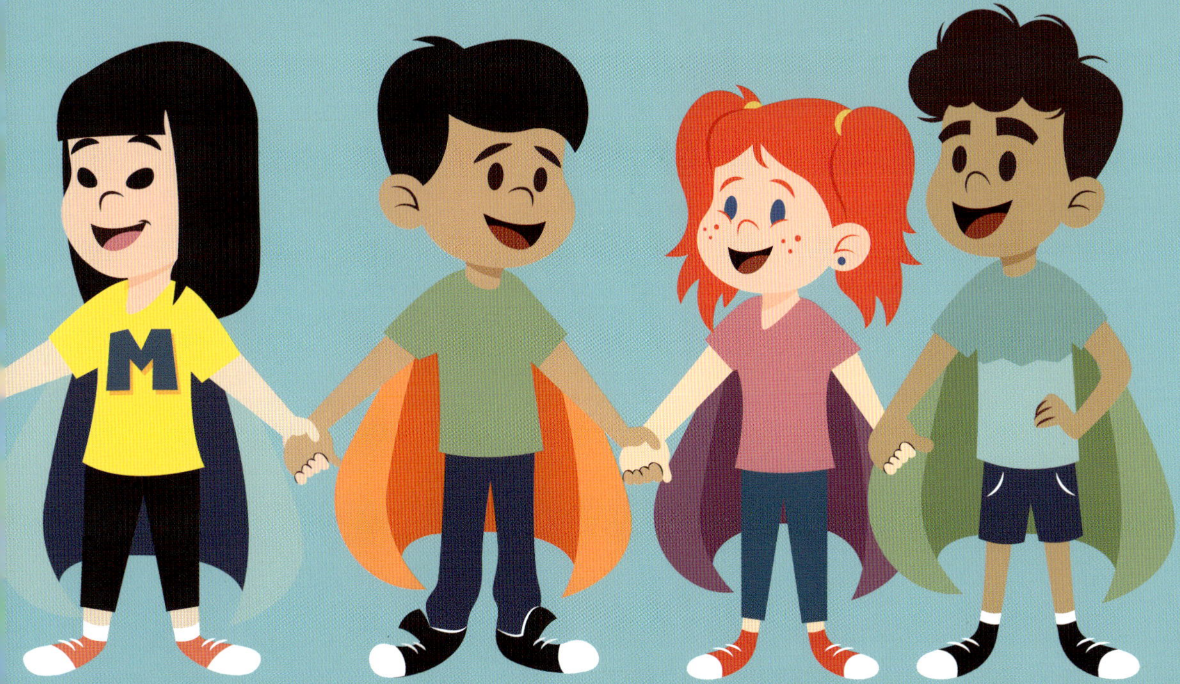

How would you describe mindfulness to a friend?

What is one way you could use mindfulness today?

for **PARENTS, EDUCATORS,** *and* **CAREGIVERS**

Mindfulness Superpower Practice!

Tips and Activities to Help Kids Cultivate Calm and Find Focus

Confronting new experiences is a big part of being a kid. Growing up isn't easy, and the power of mindfulness is key to staying confident, calm, and thoughtful through the many challenges of childhood. Not only can mastering mindfulness help kids respond sensibly to everyday conflicts and frustrations, but it can also lay the groundwork for lifelong emotional well-being. That's because mindfulness gives children the tools they need to manage stress and stay connected to their feelings—two skills that build resilience and emotional intelligence. At times, it's easier to suppress our difficult feelings than to acknowledge them, but until we experience them fully, those feelings will stick around. Mindfulness is especially valuable for children because it gives them a framework for regarding their feelings with kindness and curiosity—rather than avoidance—and in turn helps them engage comfortably with their full range of emotions.

In this section, you will find a selection of interactive mindfulness exercises designed to help children strengthen their superpowers. Doing these activities together with children is a great way for you to model mindful behavior and help kids make mindfulness an enduring habit.

Super Senses

Mindfulness can make us more aware of our environment and more perceptive of the small details we see, hear, smell, taste, and touch. Concentrating mindfully on the senses is one of the best ways to ground ourselves in the present moment and quiet the mind.

Superpower Practice

Superheroes are known for having extra strong senses. Kids can, too! Help them unlock their super senses by teaching them to pay very close attention to their surroundings. As they check in with each sense, have them focus mindfully and try to pick out as many details as possible. They might even detect some sights, sounds, tastes, or smells they never noticed before.

Discussion Questions

Look around the room. Name 10 of the tiniest details you can see.

Now focus on your ears by listening. What is the quietest sound you hear?

Name three things you can feel with your sense of touch. How do they feel different?

Take a slow, deep breath, in through your nose and out through your mouth. Did you notice any smells?

Try to find at least two feelings or sensations inside your body, such as anger, calm, butterflies in your stomach, or tight muscles.

Superhero Stance

Our bodies are closely connected to our emotions. That's why scanning our bodies for areas that feel tense can help us relax and changing our posture can make us feel more self-assured. This activity is all about learning how your brain and body can work together to feel calm and confident.

Superpower Practice

Have the child imagine they are a powerful superhero, like Ming did. Have them pick a superhero name and picture the perfect costume. Now, ask them to place their hands on their hips and plant their feet firmly on the ground. Tell them to pull their shoulders back and stretch their neck out as they stand tall and proud. Encourage them to think of a time they felt strong on the inside.

Discussion Questions

How does your body feel when you are scared or worried?

How does your body feel when you are proud and confident?

What are three of your best qualities?

Do your feelings change inside when you think about your strengths?

Think of one situation where your superhero stance could help you.

Flying Meditation

Though it's important to sit with our anger, sadness, and worry, we don't want to become so fixated on a single feeling that we forget to make space for our other emotions. Mindfulness can help kids keep their feelings in perspective and avoid becoming stuck on one emotion. Certain guided meditations are especially good for reconnecting with the various thoughts and feelings we all hold inside.

Superpower Practice

Have the child pretend to be a superhero flying through the sky, surrounded by fluffy white clouds. Have them imagine each cloud is a thought drifting through their mind. They can't change their thoughts or how fast they go by, so remind them to just observe. Let them know it's okay if they lose focus—just imagine new thoughts on their own clouds and go back to watching the sky.

Discussion Questions

What did your imagined clouds look like?

How fast were your imagined clouds moving?

Were the thoughts on each cloud mostly the same, or were they different?

If you got distracted from the clouds, what did you do next?

If you were flying through the sky, what would you see, hear, feel, and smell?

Super Calm Jar

Make your own Super Calm Jar by finding a bottle or jar and filling 75 percent of it with water and 15 percent of it with clear glue. Leave the remaining 10 percent empty. Gradually add superfine glitter and other optional items like confetti or beads. Once you're happy with how the mixture looks, secure the lid with glue or duct tape. You'll find that racing thoughts and worries settle as you mindfully watch the glitter flutter and fall.

Superpower Practice

First, have the child shake up the jar, imagining the swirling specks of glitter are feelings, thoughts, or worries they have. Then, have them hold the jar still, focusing mindfully on watching the glitter fall. Remind them that there is nothing they can do to change the glitter or make it sink faster. Have them simply concentrate on what they see in the jar until it stops swirling.

Discussion Questions

What makes your thoughts swirl?

What helps your thoughts settle?

How do you feel when your mind is shaken up?

What are three things you noticed about your Super Calm Jar while it was settling?

Did your thoughts or feelings change while the glitter was sinking?

Superhero Coping Kits

For coping skills to work in stressful situations, children need to practice them when they are calm. The Superhero Coping Kit is a toolbox for kids to store items related to their coping skills, including relaxation scripts, journals, or objects that stimulate the senses with unique textures or qualities. Decorating the kit with superhero designs will help kids stay interested in exercising their skills.

Superpower Practice

Find an empty box. Provide art supplies for the child to decorate the box. Next, think about mindful coping skills and have them gather up any items that can help them stay grounded in the moment, such as textured toys, affirmation and relaxation scripts, and journals. Put everything they've gathered into the box. Have them open it up whenever they have a chance to practice their superpowers.

Discussion Questions

Which object in your kit is most interesting to touch? What does it feel like?

How do you know when it's time to use a coping skill?

Which coping skills do you use when you're feeling angry?

Which coping skills work best for you?

Which coping skills do you need to practice more?

Superhero Progressive Muscle Relaxation

Progressive muscle relaxation (PMR) relieves physical tension through tightening certain muscles and then releasing them. Because it can bring mindful attention to various parts of the body, PMR can be especially helpful for getting children who have low body awareness to relax their muscles. This is a superhero twist on PMR.

Superpower Practice

Have the child reach their arms up over their head, as if they are a superhero blasting off. Now, have them dangle their arms by their sides like a cape. Have them make fists as tight as they can to show off their super strength; then have them open their hands and wiggle their fingers. Next, have them tighten their stomach muscles to make them hard like steel before relaxing and feeling their belly jiggle. Continue to have them practice tightening and relaxing the muscles in their shoulders, arms, legs, and feet.

Discussion Questions

How can you tell when your body needs to relax?

How did it feel to tighten your muscles? How did it feel to relax your muscles?

Are any muscles still tight when you scan your body? If so, squeeze and relax those muscles again.

How does your body feel now?

Super Shield or Cape

Children who are aware of their strengths tend to feel more confident and prepared to face life's challenges. In this activity, the child will create a shield or cape featuring decorations that represent their most positive attributes and supportive relationships.

Superpower Practice

Help the child shape a shield or cape out of cardboard, paper, fabric, yarn, or other available materials. Use markers to divide it into four parts. In one section, have them draw or write about their personality strengths. In the next section, have them illustrate or paste photos of the people who support them most. In the third section, have them describe coping tools they've learned in this book, and in the fourth section, have them list or draw things they are good at.

Discussion Questions

What are three things you like best about yourself?

What are three things your family or friends like about you?

What was the last coping skill you used to face a challenge?

What compliment do you most like to receive?

What is your proudest accomplishment?

Resources

***Be Mindful of Monsters* by Lauren Stockly**
This is a story about using mindfulness to accept uncomfortable emotions, paired with the *Mindful Monsters Therapeutic Workbook*, a collection of interactive exercises.

CognitiveLeap.com
Cognitive Leap incorporates mindfulness into programs and technology to help children manage emotional and cognitive challenges.

CreativePlayTherapist.com
Creative Play Therapist is a blog that provides child therapists with free resources and interventions.

JoinHopscotch.com/hopscotch-family
Hopscotch is an online platform that offers services and resources for families and mental health professionals.

LianaLowenstein.com
Liana Lowenstein is a leading child therapist, and her website includes resources for therapists and parents.

Mindful.org
Mindful is a website for parents and therapists that promotes the practice of mindfulness in blog posts and trainings.

***Mindful Parenting* by Kristen Race**
Mindful Parenting helps children (and their parents) feel happier, healthier, and calmer.

PalouseMindfulness.com
Palouse Mindfulness offers a free eight-week online course of mindfulness-based stress reduction (MBSR) training for adults.

UCLAHealth.org/marc/ucla-mindful-app
UCLA Mindful is a free app for all ages featuring guided meditations in more than a dozen languages.

Acknowledgments

This book would not have been possible without the influence of a few important individuals.

To my clients: Your brightness and creativity never cease to amaze me. You are the inspiration that keeps me striving to develop new therapeutic tools—including this book!

To my loving partner (and editor), Joe Rihn: Thank you for always helping me find the right words.

To Wendy Ludecke Selevitch: Thank you for all you've done for me in my career as a clinician and beyond. Your generosity and support make all the difference.

About the Author

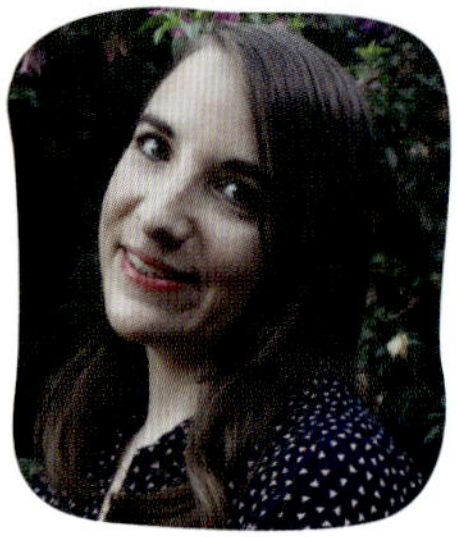

Lauren Stockly, LCSW, RPT-S, ECMHS, PPSC, is a Los Angeles-based child and adolescent mental health therapist who specializes in using play therapy to treat trauma and support emotional growth for children and families. In addition to her practice, Lauren runs the popular *Creative Play Therapist* blog and is the clinical director of Cognitive Leap, where she designs therapeutic games and programs. She is also the author of the award-winning children's book *Be Mindful of Monsters* and founder of Bumble BLS, a line of kid-friendly tools that help soothe the nervous system.

About the Illustrator

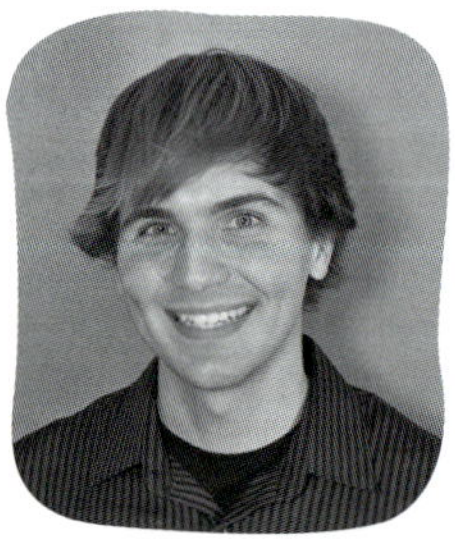

Zach Grzeszkowiak is a graphic designer and illustrator originally from the Chicagoland area. He creates both digital and printed marketing materials like logos, info-graphics, and catalogs. In addition to his responsibilities as a designer, Zach also enjoys illustrating, animating, and sculpting colorful and exciting characters. His favorite types of projects to work on involve educating, storytelling, and promoting positive change.

What *Superpower* Will You Learn Next?

Get the whole series and
explore more skills that make kids super.

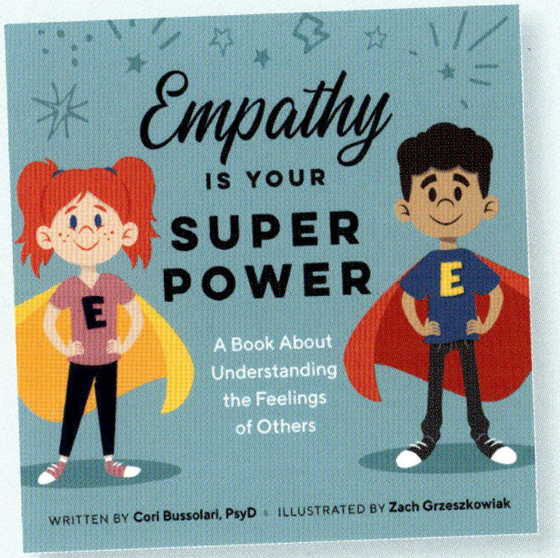

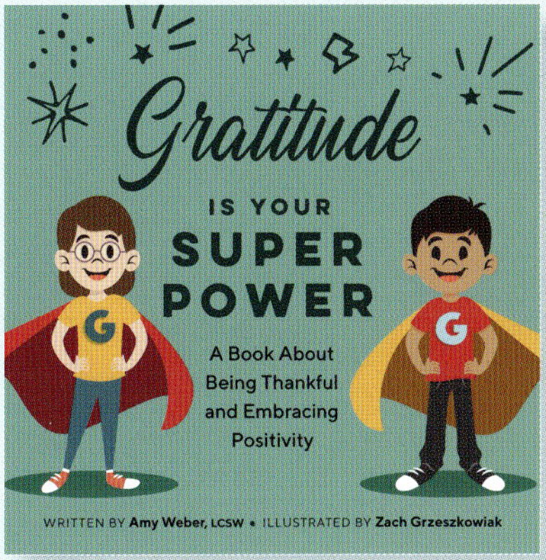

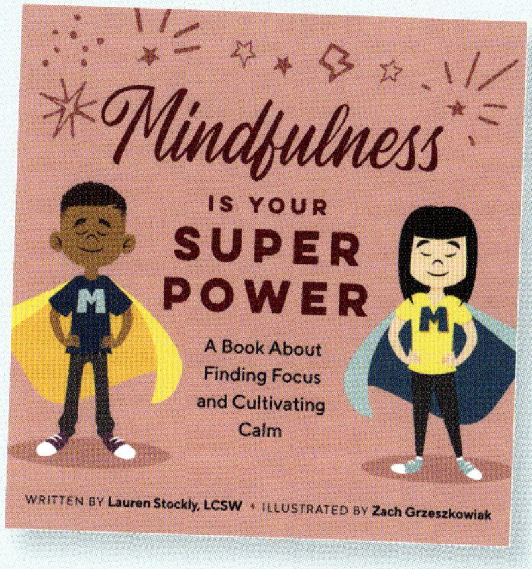

Look for this series wherever books and ebooks are sold.

DISCOVER THE POWER OF FEELINGS

Empathy Is Your Superpower
Gratitude Is Your Superpower
Confidence Is Your Superpower
Mindfulness Is Your Superpower

SHOW THEM THE POWER OF STAYING IN THE MOMENT

AN INTRODUCTION TO SELF-CONFIDENCE FOR KIDS 5 TO 7

Learning awareness and acceptance of your feelings and surroundings is an important step in growing up—and it's never too early to start. This beautifully illustrated storybook teaches young kids how to be curious and resilient in the face of challenges through real-life scenarios that are easy for them to understand. It's written with clear language for adults to read aloud and features discussion questions and activities that encourage kids to talk about what they learned and use those skills every day.

MINDFULNESS HEROES
Little superheroes Ming and Mateo model easy, age-appropriate ways for kids to be more mindful every day.

SETTING A GOOD EXAMPLE
Kids will learn how to let go of stress and anger, organize their thoughts before reacting, and inspire others to focus on the here and now.

BEYOND THIS BOOK
These tips, reflections, and games will help kids create mindfulness habits they can use for the rest of their lives.

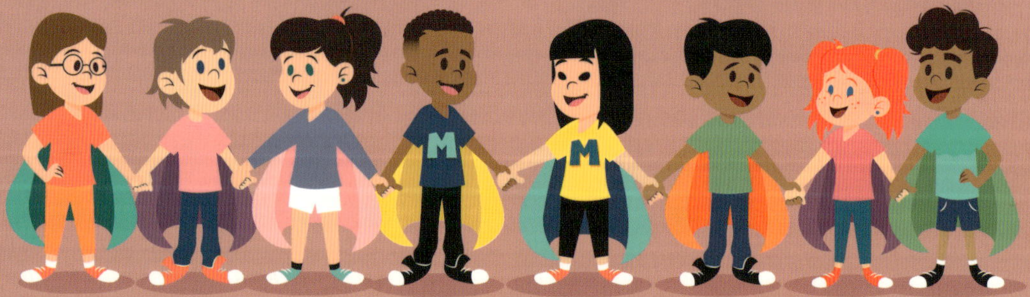

U.S. $7.99 CAN $10.99 RO
ISBN 978-1-63878-399-2
50799
9 781638 783992
WWW.ROCKRIDGEPRESS.COM

LAUREN STOCKLY, LCSW, RPT-S, ECMHS, PPSC, is an author and child therapist who specializes in using play therapy to treat trauma and support emotional growth for children and families.

Gratitude IS YOUR SUPER POWER

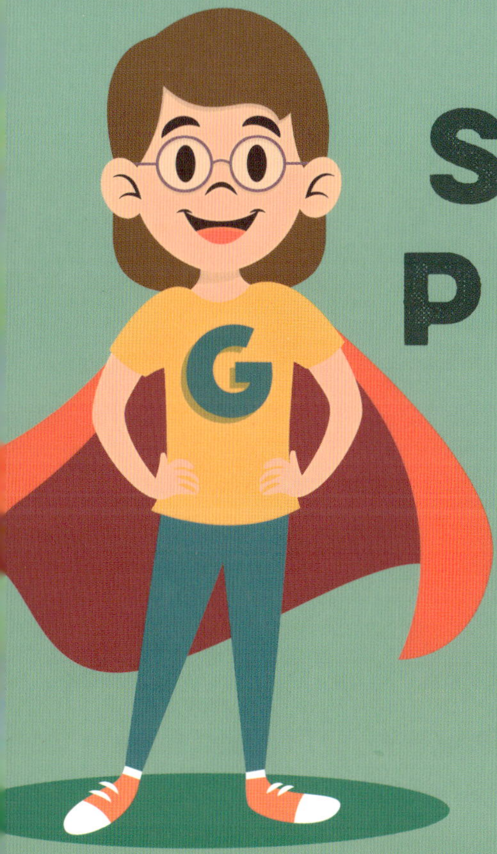

A Book About Being Thankful and Embracing Positivity

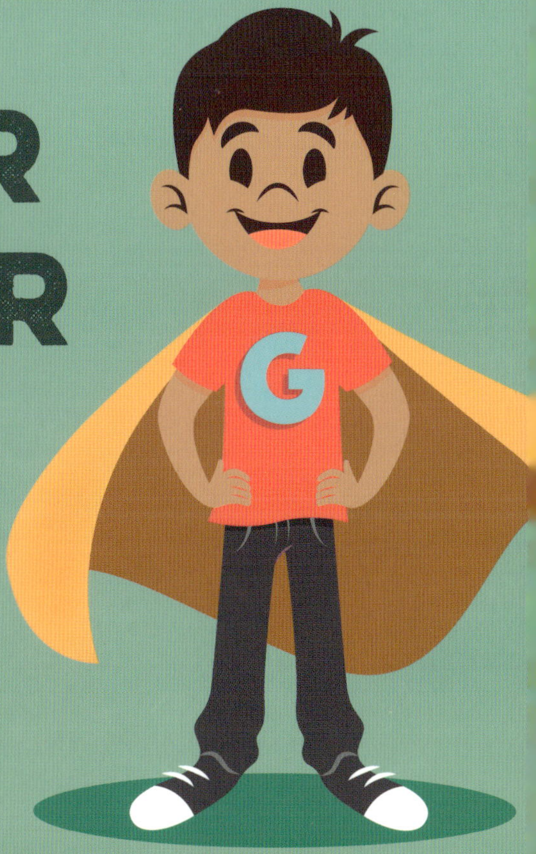

WRITTEN BY **Amy Weber,** LCSW • ILLUSTRATED BY **Zach Grzeszkowiak**